# Table of Contents

# CHAPTER 1

## INTRODUCTION

A depressed person is not abnormal but just needs help to overcome the condition. Depression can be a lonely illness and help and support from family and friends can bring about life changing and life lasting results.

There are various situations in life where an individual may have to go through the procedure of depression. Although the cause of depression varies from person to person, the main reason may be due to some personal problems which may be work related, relationship problems or due to family problems but personal and family problems mainly contribute to the build up of depression.

For many, depression does not seem complex because they live with it. But depression causes problems in work, social life, family adjustment. If you suffer from depression then you must be well aware of the problems that you face, but it is not only you that suffer, but people around you suffer too because they care for you.

### What Is Depression?

Depression is an illness that affects your brain. It is your reaction to something sad, loss of someone, or dejection. When these feelings aggravate and become intense, it leads to a medical condition called clinical depression.

**Symptoms Of Depression**

- You feel worthless and guilty on a daily basis
- Your concentration decreases and indecisiveness takes over
- All the hobbies and activities you enjoyed previously now don't seem appealing at all
- You think about death and contemplate suicide
- You feel unstable and fidgety or incredibly dull and slow
- There will be a significant change in your weight – you either gain it or lose it

**Causes of Depression**

When you get emotionally attached to something over a period, and it doesn't exist anymore, it leaves a gap, and depression takes over to cope with the loss. Genetics, fluctuation in the hormone levels, some medical conditions, post-surgery reaction, and high stress levels also cause depression. It is a common yet severe problem that needs to be tackled before it gets out of hand. Let's now find out how yoga and depression are related.

**Types of Depression**

You may wonder how can there be different types of depression. The truth is that there are 5 types of depressions and the following section explains it further.

- *Major Depression:* This is the most serious type and the variety and number of symptoms are huge.
- *Dysthymic Disorder:* A depression that is generally moderate and has been present for nearly two years or at times longer.
- *Unspecified Depression:* This type exists in people who have depression that is quite serious in nature but not severe in nature.
- *Adjustment Disorder Depression:* A type of depression that occurs with people due to problems or due to a crisis in one's life.
- *Bipolar Depression:* People facing this type of depression may have low and high mood swings along with other symptoms.

If you suffer from depression, this book "Depression Therapy" will help you to combat it. You can do depression therapy on your own and the first thing you need to do is stop thinking negative. Negative thinking is the main reason for depression and it pulls any person back from achieving what they want to do. The following steps given below are useful when considering a good depression therapy and will be further discussed in consecutive chapters:

- *Yoga,*
- *Exercises, and*
- *Natural food.*

**Other Depression Treatment Options**

Just as there are many types of depression, there are also various depression treatment options that are tailored to help alleviate or resolve depressive disorders. The more common ways to treat these disorders are with medications, therapy, counseling, self help approaches and intense hospitalization in severe cases. There are various alternatives to these approaches as well that are often applied that can be successful depending upon the particular situation.

- *Medications:* Traditional medications include antidepressants, anti-anxiety medications and other mood stabilizers that are often prescribed to those who suffer with depression. Each medication is quite different and may not work on every person, so sometimes it is a trial and error experiment to find the best medication that works for certain symptoms.

  Most patients will use a medication for a few weeks to monitor results and then switch to another if needed for a more positive outcome. These types of medications can alleviate some of the more severe emotional feelings such as sadness, hopelessness and suicidal thoughts. The right medication can provide a mild emotional lift while a patient is working through the root causes of a depressive disorder.

- *Therapy:* There are various types of therapies used to help dissipate the worst of depressive symptoms. Light therapy and electroshock therapy (ECT) have been used for years when needed as part of various treatment plans. Specific recreational and exercise therapies are also recommended to people who suffer from depression.

- ***Counseling:*** Professional counseling structured by a psychiatrist, professional counselor, pastor or other mental health provider is a very important ingredient in the recovery process for many people. Counseling can be used alone or as part of an overall treatment process in helping resolve a depressive problem.

- ***Self Help:*** Many people benefit greatly from books, community groups, church support groups, online communities and other avenues of self help approaches that target various issues associated with depression. Self help approaches can be extremely positive and help a struggling person find personal balance and healing sometimes without additional assistance.

- ***Alternative Approaches:*** There are various experimental treatments that are on the horizon or are already in use on a small scale that are producing promising results. One approach uses high powered magnets applied to the skull that actually alters mood for those who are extremely depressed. It is applied with no medication or other accompanying applications and without pain. In a small sampling of people so far, it has proved highly beneficial. Natural alternatives for depression are of especial interest to many people.

# CHAPTER 2

## YOGA THERAPY

Yoga is one of the best ways to lighten your mood and keep depression at bay. Yoga poses increase blood circulation to the brain and enable the production of the mood-elevating hormones.

The practice of yoga doesn't have any adverse side effects, which make it a better option as compared to other medication for depression. Some yoga poses to fight depression are mentioned below. Try them for at least 12 weeks to notice significant changes.

Yoga is a physical exercise that involves different body poses, breathing techniques, and meditation. The therapy may help with depression and your symptoms, such as difficulty concentrating or loss of energy.

Many people use yoga therapy to manage:

- mental and emotional problems, such as stress, anxiety, or depression
- conditions and disorders, such as ongoing low back pain
- chronic or long-term pain
- overall health and well-being

You can find yoga classes at fitness studios, hospitals, and local community centers. The classes can be gentle or challenging, depending on the style.

**The 5 Best Yoga Poses For Depression**

To offer you this article for free we receive a small affiliate commission if you chose to buy through our links. Click here to learn more.

Depression is one of the most common and devastating mental health problems that people face today.

1. Bridge Pose (Sethu Bandhasana)
2. Downward-Facing Dog Pose (Adho Mukha Svanasana)
3. Child Pose (Balasana)
4. Cobra Pose (Bhujangasana)
5. Corpse Pose (Shavasana)

Depression doesn't distinguish between rich or poor, old or young: nearly everyone is susceptible.It can decrease your energy levels, interest in work and hobbies, severely harm your relationships, and lead to low quality of life.

Let's face it. Americans are one of the most over-prescribed cultures in the history of mankind.

And when it comes to treatment of depression, the outlook is dim. Whether it be SSRIs like Prozac or stimulants like Provigil, there's no shortage of drugs designed to 'make us happy'.

While appropriate medical treatments are sometimes necessary in the management of depression, other practices like meditation and yoga can also help lessen the effects that depression has upon the body and mind.

As with any method of combating a depressive disorder, consistency is key; make sure you stick with your yoga routine for a few months in order to reap the full benefits of your practice. Take your time, and fully immerse yourself in the poses for maximum effectiveness.

Studies have indicated that practicing yoga helps to modulate the body's stress response systems, consequently lessening some of the symptoms of depression. Yoga can also give your mood a boost and improve your ability to function and motivate yourself.

Yoga can calm and focus the mind, helping to soothe your mood and divert your attention away from negative thoughts. Let's take a look at some of the best yoga poses for easing and managing the symptoms of depression.

**Bridge Pose (Sethu Bandhasana)**

The Bridge Pose is a good one for easing anxiety and mental stress, since it engages the spine, neck, and hips. Poor alignment can worsen your mood by placing added strain upon the nerves in the back and shoulders, which in turn can have negative effects upon your ability to manage anxiety disorders.

To begin forming the Bridge Pose, lie flat on your back with your palms facing down.

Bend your knees and rest your feet flat on the floor, bringing your feet as close to your buttocks as you can. Pay attention to your body's limitations, and do not force any stretch to the point of straining your knees or other joints.

Inhale and lift your hips off the floor. Bring your hands to meet underneath your body and lace your fingers together.

Press down through your feet, arms, and shoulders to lift your hips further. Tense your inner thighs for support and aim to point your tailbone straight towards your knees.

Hold this position for five to seven breaths. Exhale as you slowly and carefully lower your hips back down to the floor and release the posture.

**Downward-Facing Dog Pose (Adho Mukha Svanasana)**

The Downward-Facing Dog Pose will help counteract the feelings of heaviness and fatigue that often come with depression.

This pose engages many different areas of the body, stretching them out and resulting in a more relaxed state. The neck and back in particular are engaged while practicing this pose, which increases blood flow and relaxes the areas of the body where people often carry their stress.

Begin on your hands and knees, with your knees separated as widely as your hips and your legs and feet pointing straight back. Your hands should meet the floor directly under your shoulders, with your fingers spread wide for the best stability.

Walk your hands just slightly forward so that they're in front of your shoulders, and then curl your toes under.

Push up through your legs to lift your sitting bones upwards and straighten your legs as much as possible without locking them. Keeping the joints supple while going through your yoga routine is very important.

Draw your shoulder blades together and lower your chest. Your ears should line up with your arms, your spine should be straight, and your body should form an inverted "V" shape.

Hold this pose for five to seven breaths, then slowly bend your legs and exhale as you descend back to your hands and knees.

**Child Pose (Balasana)**

One of the most comfortable and relaxing yoga poses, the Child Pose provides a gentle stretch of the lower back and hip area. Practicing this pose can help relax and improve the alignment of your back, helping you decompress and easing your negative feelings.

Child Pose helps you to relax and release tension from your shoulders and upper torso, which are areas where people commonly carry their stress. Softening these areas of the body can help lessen the physical burden of depression.

To begin this pose, start in a kneeling position with your knees hip width apart. Bring your feet together so that your big toes touch one another.

Bend forward so that your torso lays down between your thighs, and reach your arms forward to rest the palms of your hands flat on the floor.

Point your tailbone back and away from your pelvic area to stretch and straighten your spine. Settle your weight more completely onto your thighs.

Let your forehead rest on the floor and relax your body. Let the weight of your arms gently spread your shoulder blades apart.

Child Pose is a "resting pose", so you can stay in this position for longer than you can hold the more active poses several minutes if you like. When you are finished, bring your hands beneath your shoulders and slowly push up into a kneeling position to avoid straining your back.

## Cobra Pose (Bhujangasana)

The Cobra Pose focuses on increasing flexibility in the spine, as well as opening and stretching the chest area of the torso. Since many people carry depressive feelings in the chest and back, stretching and releasing tension in these places can help to lessen some of the symptoms of depression and lift your mood.

To begin the Cobra Pose, lie face-down on the floor with your legs extended behind you. Do not curl your toes; rest the tops of your feet on the floor instead.

Place your hands below your shoulders with your fingers spread wide and your palms pressed firmly into the floor. Keep your elbows very close to the sides of your body.

Press down through the tops of your feet and your pubic bone, as well as through your hands. Inhale deeply and lift your chest and head away from the floor. Keep your pelvic area connected with the floor to ensure that you're getting the best possible back bend.

Pull your shoulders back to open your chest. Make sure you keep your shoulders dropped away from your ears to keep from scrunching or tensing your neck. If you are less flexible, look at the floor or straight ahead. If you feel ready to explore a deeper bend, lift your gaze towards the sky.

**Corpse Pose (Shavasana)**

The Corpse Pose is often used to finish off a yoga session in order to encourage your body to more fully absorb the benefits of your practice. It is the state of complete relaxation, both in mind and in body, and can do wonders to help ease feelings of depression and anxiety.

The full-body relaxation of this pose can provide you with an energy boost after its completion, which can be invaluable in the face of depression. Shavasana poses also have a ton of added health benefits for pregnant moms.

To begin the Corpse Pose, lie flat on your back. Let your arms rest slightly away from the sides of your body where they feel most natural, and let the palms of your hands face upwards.

Let your feet rest at a comfortable width apart (many people prefer hip width), and allow your feet to naturally turn outwards.

Slowly begin to guide your focus to each part of your body, beginning with your feet and moving up through the various areas of your body. While you focus, breathe very slowly and deeply, willing each part of your body to relax.

Move through each part of your body, breathing deeply and relaxing the area you're focusing on each time you exhale.

Take your time, and surrender fully to the experience of being completely relaxed. Take care to maintain your mental focus and do not let yourself doze off.

After around ten minutes, when you have completed the process of relaxing your entire body and taking in the state of calmness, keep your eyes closed and roll to one side. Let your body curl gently if it feels natural, and rest there for a minute.

When you are ready, push your hand against the floor to carefully lift your body into a sitting position.

**Why Use Yoga as a Adjunct Treatment for Depression?**

Depression is such a varied and complex illness that a "one size fits all" approach is unlikely to be fully effective for a significant proportion of patients. People with depression often have to weigh up the benefits of antidepressants with their well-reported side effects. Unfortunately, the fact that depression is still far from being entirely understood means that there is no perfect solution.

Within the context of pharmaceutical and other therapeutic remedies, yoga therapy can assist people in symptom management and recovery and in cases of mild depression, it can be their primary self-help tool which prevents their symptoms from worsening.

People with depression exhibit elevated levels of cortisol, which is related to brain changes in the hippocampus, prefrontal cortex and amygdala. While the hippocampus and prefrontal cortex (which are involved in emotion regulation, memory forming and decision making) appear to lose volume, the amygdala (responsible for our fear and stress response) becomes enlarged and more active. Known as the "stress hormone", those with depression exhibit greater cortisol levels at all points during the day than people without depression.

Studies have demonstrated reduced levels of cortisol in those who practice yoga. It's thought that the breathing exercises that are a key part of yoga induce the body's relaxation response, and mindfulness meditation (another aspect of yoga) is also associated with lowering cortisol in study subjects as well as reductions in the size of the amygdala. In one study, participants exhibited lower cortisol levels immediately after a yoga class – which suggests the effect isn't confined to long-term practice.

Depression also appears to be linked to reduced levels of certain GABA neurotransmitters, with "increasing evidence points to an association between major depressive disorders (MDDs) and diverse types of GABAergic deficits." A 12-week yoga intervention found greater improvements in mood than a metabolically matched walking exercise, and also was "the first time that yoga postures have been associated with a positive correlation between acute increases in thalamic GABA levels".

One promising study showed a reduction in suicide ideation for people suffering with depression after 12-week yoga intervention, concluding (while further studies are needed) that Iyengar yoga is a safe intervention for those whose symptoms include suicide ideation without intent.

Another benefit of yoga is that it offers a form of exercise to people living with or prone to depression. The efficacy of exercise for decreasing symptoms of depression has been well established and given that depression is known to drain motivation, yoga can offer a gentle and enjoyable way to begin a exercise regime. Yoga is a non-judgemental practice that is beneficial to people whatever their "skill" level, and yoga classes are welcoming spaces that can provide a supportive sense of community.

This is important for people living with depression, as feelings of worthlessness and self-blame might be a barrier to physical activity. Another barrier is the experience of depression itself. When someone is suffering with a severe depressive episode they may find it hard to even leave their bed, wash or eat, so it would be unrealistic to expect them to attend a yoga class. It is therefore important to suggest a yoga intervention at an appropriate time, where the practice will aid in recovery and help to prevent a major resurgence of symptoms.

**Pros and Cons of Yoga Therapy**

Yoga complements traditional therapies, such as medication and psychotherapy. But it's not meant to be a sole treatment.

*Yoga is;*

- generally safe when practiced properly
- beneficial for people who want to improve concentration
- available in many styles for all levels

*Yoga can be;*

- challenging for beginners and people with limited flexibility
- uncomfortable, depending on the pose
- expensive, depending on the studio

Studies show that yoga therapy can help with stress, anxiety, and depression. Yoga is a gentle exercise that incorporates both meditation and controlled, physical movements. The focus on deep breathing and stretching your body is effective for relieving the symptoms of depression, such as sleep troubles, pain, and a loss of energy.

No matter which style of yoga you choose, you can adapt the poses to suit your level.

Many studios, hospitals, and local community centers offer yoga classes. But yoga can be expensive, especially if you want to practice every day. Thankfully, many instructional videos are available online, such as on YouTube, and through apps.

# CHAPTER 3

## EXERCISING

Being depressed can leave you feeling low in energy, which might put you off being more active.

Regular exercise can boost your mood if you have depression, and it's especially useful for people with mild to moderate depression.

*"Exercise should be something you enjoy; otherwise, it will be hard to find the motivation to do it regularly."*

When you have depression or anxiety, exercise often seems like the last thing you want to do. But once you get motivated, exercise can make a big difference.

Exercise helps prevent and improve a number of health problems, including high blood pressure, diabetes and arthritis. Research on depression, anxiety and exercise shows that the psychological and physical benefits of exercise can also help improve mood and reduce anxiety.

The links between depression, anxiety and exercise aren't entirely clear but working out and other forms of physical activity can definitely ease symptoms of depression or anxiety and make you feel better. Exercise may also help keep depression and anxiety from coming back once you're feeling better.

**How Exercise Help Depression**

**Regular exercise may help ease depression by:**

- Releasing feel-good endorphins, natural cannabis-like brain chemicals (endogenous cannabinoids) and other natural brain chemicals that can enhance your sense of well-being
- Taking your mind off worries so you can get away from the cycle of negative thoughts that feed depression and anxiety

**Regular exercise has many psychological and emotional benefits, too. It can help you:**

*Gain confidence.* Meeting exercise goals or challenges, even small ones, can boost your self-confidence. Getting in shape can also make you feel better about your appearance.

*Get more social interaction.* Exercise and physical activity may give you the chance to meet or socialize with others. Just exchanging a friendly smile or greeting as you walk around your neighborhood can help your mood.

*Cope in a healthy way.* Doing something positive to manage depression or anxiety is a healthy coping strategy. Trying to feel better by drinking alcohol, dwelling on how you feel, or hoping depression or anxiety will go away on its own can lead to worsening symptoms.

**Added Benefits Of Exercise**

Each of us has different amounts of neurotransmitters and endorphins in circulation. These are strongly affected by both nutrition and physical activity. Additionally, exercise reduces immune system chemicals that can exacerbate depression.

Along with the physical and psychological effects of exercise, a structured exercise program helps those with depression by giving purpose and structure to the day. Exercising outdoors comes with the added advantage of being exposed to sunlight, which affects our pineal glands, boosting our moods.

**Planning An Exercise Program**

If you or someone you know is suffering from depression, it is important to plan an exercise program that will work. Make sure the forms of exercise are enjoyable, and factor in more than one, if possible, as variety is the spice of life. Set some achievable goals and decide if you prefer to exercise in a group situation, by yourself or with an exercise partner. Many people find it helps to have a partner or group as part of their plan, to get support and to continue to feel motivated. Exercise logs can also be helpful, as a way of monitoring your progress.

**How Often Do You Need To Exercise?**

To stay healthy, adults should do 150 minutes of moderate-intensity activity every week.

If you haven't exercised for a while, start gradually and aim to build up towards acheiving 150 minutes a week.

Any exercise is better than none. Even a brisk 10-minute walk can clear your mind and help you relax.

**How do I get started and stay motivated?**

Starting and sticking with an exercise routine or regular physical activity can be a challenge. These steps can help:

- ***Identify what you enjoy doing.*** Figure out what type of physical activities you're most likely to do, and think about when and how you'd be most likely to follow through. For instance, would you be more likely to do some gardening in the evening, start your day with a jog, or go for a bike ride or play basketball with your children after school? Do what you enjoy to help you stick with it.

- ***Get your mental health professional's support.*** Talk to your doctor or mental health professional for guidance and support. Discuss an exercise program or physical activity routine and how it fits into your overall treatment plan.

- ***Set reasonable goals.*** Your mission doesn't have to be walking for an hour five days a week. Think realistically about what you may be able to do and begin gradually. Tailor your plan to your own needs and abilities rather than setting unrealistic guidelines that you're unlikely to meet.

- ***Don't think of exercise or physical activity as a chore.*** If exercise is just another "should" in your life that you don't think you're living up to, you'll associate it with failure. Rather, look at your exercise or physical activity schedule the same way you look at your therapy sessions or medication as one of the tools to help you get better.

- ***Analyze your barriers.*** Figure out what's stopping you from being physically active or exercising. If you feel self-conscious, for instance, you may want to exercise at home. If you stick to goals better with a partner, find a friend to work out with or who enjoys the same physical activities that you do. If you don't have money to spend on exercise gear, do something that's cost-free, such as regular walking. If you think about what's stopping you from being physically active or exercising, you can probably find an alternative solution.

- ***Prepare for setbacks and obstacles.*** Give yourself credit for every step in the right direction, no matter how small. If you skip exercise one day, that doesn't mean you can't maintain an exercise routine and might as well quit. Just try again the next day. Stick with it.

## 7 Great Exercises To Ease Depression

Exercise may trigger feel-good chemicals in your brain and help eliminate symptoms of depression so get moving!

Break a Sweat for Depression Relief: Could a trip to the gym be just what the therapist ordered?

Exercise certainly isn't a depression cure-all, but a study published in the Journal of Sport and Exercise Psychology found that heart-pumping, endorphin-boosting workouts actually promote happiness.

Researchers say that more physically active people reported greater general feelings of excitement and enthusiasm than less-active people. And beyond its protective effect against feelings of depression, exercise may reduce stress and help you secure a better night's sleep. That's why your favorite fitness routine can be an excellent addition to your depression treatment plan.

Exercise stimulates the release of many of the brain chemicals thought to be in low supply when someone is battling depression.

**Set Off That Runner's High:** When it comes to workouts that fight depression, aerobic and cardio exercises have the edge. "To date, the strongest evidence seems to support aerobic exercise. While the correct "dose" of depression-fighting exercise is up for debate, some experts recommend 20 to 30 minutes most days of the week. A recent review of numerous scientific studies found no association between the intensity level of the exercise and its emotional benefit so simply moving more is a great start.

Ever heard of runner's high? The most tangible example of exercise stimulating certain brain chemicals is the runner's high that many athletes report experiencing once crossing a certain threshold of exertion while running. That euphoria is due to the release of endorphins in the brain in response to the sustained physical activity.

Endorphins are our body's natural morphine and, when released by special glands in our brains, they can produce a sense of well-being or joy and also decrease pain levels.

**Build Your Muscles:** Boost your strength, boost your happiness? A recent study of 45 stroke survivors with depression found that a 10-week strength training program helped reduced symptoms of depression (among numerous other benefits).

Strength training is about mastery and control, it requires full attention and concentration. More importantly, people can see the results, the outline of the muscles forming, from dedication and training.

Just be sure to start slowly and use the assistance of a personal trainer if needed.

**Become a Yogi:** Ohm — in a study of 65 women with depression and anxiety, the 34 women who took a yoga class twice a week for two months showed a significant decrease in depression and anxiety symptoms, compared to the 31 women who were not in the class.

Eastern traditions such as yoga have a wonderful antidepressant effect in that they improve flexibility; involve mindfulness, which breaks up repetitive negative thoughts; increase strength; make you aware of your breathing; improve balance; and contain a meditative component.

**Try Tai Chi:** Like yoga, the slow, gentle movements of tai chi are another Eastern tradition that might help you break free from depression or major depressive disorder.

In a study of 14 older Chinese patients with depression, those who took tai chi over a three-month period showed a significant improvement in their depression symptoms. The researchers theorized that the social aspects of tai chi, which is done in group settings, may have also played a role in its effectiveness.

**Get Your Walk On:** Simply putting one foot in front of the other may be the trick to feeling better that's because walking is an aerobic exercise that's suited for almost everyone. All it takes is a pair of comfortable, supportive shoes, and you're ready to go.

Practical wisdom suggests that doing something is better than doing nothing in terms of physical activity. If depression has made you sedentary, start off slowly and gradually increase time and distance.

**Go Play Outside:** If you enjoy being outdoors, even simple activities such as gardening, throwing a ball around with your kids, or washing your car may do you some good. That's because a healthy dose of sunlight has been shown to boost mood, likely due to the fact that sunshine stimulates our serotonin levels (drops in serotonin during the darker, colder months have been linked to seasonal affective disorder, or SAD).

Just moving your body inside or out is exercise. Choose whatever works for you, depending on your functioning level, energy, and preferences.

**Bounce:** Want something super-simple to break you out of a funk at least temporarily? Be bouncey.

You don't need to jump, but bend your knees and bounce as quickly as you can for a few minutes. This is an easy way to oxygenate your brain and get some endorphins flowing.

**The Exercise Effect**

Exercising starts a biological cascade of events that results in many health benefits, such as protecting against heart disease and diabetes, improving sleep, and lowering blood pressure. High-intensity exercise releases the body's feel-good chemicals called endorphins, resulting in the "runner's high" that joggers report. But for most of us, the real value is in low-intensity exercise sustained over time. That kind of activity spurs the release of proteins called neurotrophic or growth factors, which cause nerve cells to grow and make new connections. The improvement in brain function makes you feel better. In people who are depressed, neuroscientists have noticed that the hippocampus in the brain the region that helps regulate mood is smaller. Exercise supports nerve cell growth in the hippocampus, improving nerve cell connections, which helps relieve depression.

**Do I need to see my doctor?**

If you haven't exercised for a long time or are concerned about the effects of exercise on your body or health, check with your doctor before starting a new exercise program to make sure it's safe for you. Talk to your doctor to find out which activities, how much exercise and what intensity level is OK for you. Your doctor will consider any medications you take and your health conditions. He or she may also have helpful advice about getting started and staying motivated.

If you exercise regularly but depression or anxiety symptoms still interfere with your daily living, see your doctor or mental health professional. Exercise and physical activity are great ways to ease symptoms of depression or anxiety, but they aren't a substitute for talk therapy (psychotherapy) or medications.

# CHAPTER 4

## NATURAL FOOD

One of the most overlooked aspects of mental health is nutrition. Food plays a significant role in our physical health, as well as our mental and emotional health. When you are struggling with depression, it can feel a bit overwhelming to think about eating the right foods. However, some of these small changes in your diet may help to decrease your symptoms and have a positive effect on your daily life.

There is no specific diet to treat depression, but eating more of some foods and less or none of others can help some people manage their symptoms.

### Link Between Diet And Depression

One factor that may contribute to depression is a person's dietary habits, which will determine the nutrients that they consume.

A 2017 study found that the symptoms of people with moderate-to-severe depression improved when they received nutritional counseling sessions and ate a more healthful diet for 12 weeks.

The improved diet focused on fresh and whole foods that are high in nutrients. It also limited processed refined foods, sweets, and fried food, including junk food.

Depressive symptoms, including mood and anxiety, improved enough to achieve remission criteria in more than 32% of the participants.

The researchers concluded that people could help manage or improve their symptoms of depression by addressing their diet.

Our brain is part of our bodies, of course.

So anything that makes our bodies healthier fresh air, sunshine, clean water, exercise, de-stressing, vitamins and minerals, improved circulation, etc. will make our brains healthier.

Some nutrients in particular seem to be linked to brain health.

**Selenium**

Some scientists have suggested that increasing selenium intake might help improve mood and reduce anxiety, which may help make depression more manageable.

*Selenium is present in a variety of foods, including:*

- whole grains
- Brazil nuts
- some seafood
- organ meats, such as liver

**Vitamin D**

Vitamin D may help improve the symptoms of depression, according to a 2019 meta-analysis.

People obtain most of their vitamin D through sun exposure, but dietary sources are also important.

***Foods that can provide vitamin D include:***

- oily fish
- fortified dairy products
- beef liver
- egg

## Omega-3 fatty acids

The results of some studies have suggested that omega-3 fatty acids might help with depressive disorders.

However, the authors of a 2015 review concluded that more studies are necessary to confirm this.

Eating omega-3 fatty acids may reduce the risk of mood disorders and brain diseases by enhancing brain function and preserving the myelin sheath that protects nerve cells.

***Good sources of omega-3 fatty acids include:***

- cold-water fish, such as salmon, sardines, tuna, and mackerel
- flaxseed, flaxseed oil, and chia seeds
- walnuts

**Antioxidants**

Vitamins A (beta carotene), C, and E contain substances called antioxidants.

Antioxidants help remove free radicals, which are the waste products of natural bodily processes that can build up in the body.

If the body cannot eliminate enough free radicals, oxidative stress can develop. A number of health problems can result, which may include anxiety and depression.

The results of a 2012 study suggested that consuming the vitamins that provide antioxidants may reduce symptoms of anxiety in people with generalized anxiety disorder.

Fresh, plant based foods, such as berries, are good sources of antioxidants. A diet that is rich in fresh fruits and vegetables, soy, and other plant products may help reduce the stress-related symptoms of depression.

**B vitamins**

Foods containing whole grains are a good source of vitamin B-12.

Vitamins B-12 and B-9 (folate, or folic acid) help protect and maintain the nervous system, including the brain. They may help reduce the risk and symptoms of mood disorders, such as depression.

*Sources of vitamin B-12 include:*

- eggs
- meat
- poultry
- fish
- oysters
- milk
- whole grains
- some fortified cereals

*Foods that contain folate include:*

- dark leafy vegetables
- fruit and fruit juices
- nuts
- beans
- whole grains
- dairy products
- meat and poultry
- seafood
- eggs

## Zinc

Zinc helps the body perceive taste, but it also boosts the immune system and may influence depression.

Some studies have suggested that zinc levels may be lower in people with depression and that zinc supplementation may help antidepressants work more effectively.

***Zinc is present in:***

- whole grains
- oysters
- beef, chicken, and pork
- beans
- nuts and pumpkin seeds

**Protein**

Protein enables the body to grow and repair, but it may also help people with depression.

The body uses a protein called tryptophan to create serotonin, the "feel good" hormone.

***Tryptophan is present in:***

- tuna
- turkey
- chickpeas

Serotonin appears to play a role in depression, but the mechanism is complex, and exactly how it works remains unclear. However, eating foods that may boost serotonin levels might be beneficial.

**Probiotics**

Foods such as yogurt and kefir may boost the levels of beneficial bacteria in the gut.

Healthy gut microbiota may reduce the symptoms and risk of depression, according to a 2016 meta-analysis. The researchers suggested that Lactobacillus and Bifidobacterium may help.

**Weight management**

Obesity appears to raise the risk of depression.

This increased risk may be due to the hormonal and immunological changes that occur in people with obesity.

A person who is overweight or has obesity may wish to consult their doctor or a dietitian about ways to manage their weight.

The Dietary Approaches to Stop Hypertension (DASH) diet, which health authorities recommend, can help reduce blood pressure and improve overall health.

There is also evidence that it can help with weight loss and may reduce the risk of depression.

**Foods to avoid**

Some foods may aggravate the symptoms of depression.

*Alcohol*

There is a clear link between alcohol and mental health problems. A person may drink as a way to cope with depression, but alcohol can aggravate or trigger new bouts of depression and anxiety.

Regularly consuming large amounts of alcohol can lead to further complications, such as accidents, family issues, loss of employment, and ill health.

Even those who limit their alcohol consumption to no more than one drink a day have a higher risk of some types of cancer, according to the National Cancer Institute. Poor health, in turn, can lead to further depression.

### *Refined foods*

Convenience foods, such as fast food and junk food, can be high in calories and low in nutrients.

Studies have suggested that people who consume lots of fast food are more likely to have depression than those who eat mostly fresh produce.

Processed foods, especially those high in sugar and refined carbs, may contribute to a higher risk of depression. When a person eats refined carbs, the body's energy levels increase rapidly but then crash. A bar of chocolate may give an instant boost, but a rapid low can follow.

It is best to opt for fresh, nutrient dense, whole foods that provide a steady source of energy over time.

### *Processed oils*

Refined and saturated fats can trigger inflammation, and they may also impair brain function and worsen the symptoms of depression.

*Fats to avoid include:*

- trans fats, which are present in many processed foods
- fats in red and processed meats
- safflower and corn oil, which are high in omega-6 fatty acids

### *Caffeine*

People with depression may benefit from not drinking caffeinated beverages after midday.

At least one study has found that a moderate intake of caffeine, in the form of coffee, may benefit people with depression. Caffeine's benefits could be due to its stimulant effect and antioxidants properties.

*Caffeine is present in:*

- coffee
- tea
- chocolate
- sodas
- energy drinks

There is some evidence that small amounts of caffeine may reduce anxiety and boost mood. However, some research has found that it may increase feelings of anxiety, stress, and depression in children of high school age.

In addition, caffeine can affect a person's ability to sleep.

***While caffeine may benefit some people, it is best to:***

- consume it only in moderation
- avoid products with a high caffeine content, such as energy drinks
- avoid caffeine after midday

**Outlook**

Diet may play a role in depression. Following a diet that is low in processed foods and provides plenty of fresh, plant-based foods and healthful fats may help improve symptoms.

***Other tips that may help include:***

- getting at least 150 minutes of physical exercise each week
- spending time outdoors
- avoiding the use of alcohol and other substances
- getting 7–8 hours of sleep in every 24 hours

A doctor can often recommend suitable treatments to help people manage the symptoms of depression, and these may include adopting a more healthful diet.

It's not as simple as just supplementing these. Nutrients work together in context. And we don't know if low levels of nutrients are a cause or consequence of poor brain health.

So you can't "biohack" your way to happiness with a few pills or "superfoods."

If you want to focus on particular nutrients and/or explore possible deficiencies, it's best to do so with a trusted health professional like a registered dietician, nutritionist or doctor trained in functional medicine.

**How Eating Right May Boost Mental Health**

Your brain is greedy. It needs a lot of energy to work properly and to create neurotransmitters chemicals that send signals through the nervous system.

Without enough energy or the right nutrients, your brain won't get what it needs. In fact, one study suggests that eating a lot of nutrient-sparse processed foods could up your chances of becoming depressed by as much as 60 percent.

Other research has shown that nutrient deficiencies often look like mental health problems.

Here are some pathways by which a healthy diet might protect your brain.

**Nutrition can fight inflammation**

Chronic inflammation happens when our body turns on an immune response, then doesn't turn it off again. The resulting damage and chemical stew is linked to all manner of health problems, including cancer, heart disease, neurodegenerative disorders like Alzheimer's… and depression.

One theory is that proinflammatory cytokines markers of inflammation may interact with other proteins in the brain, promoting changes that contribute to depressive illness.

**Nutrition can get your gut health back on track**

Your GI tract does more than move food from one end to the other. It's responsible for absorbing the nutrients your organs including the brain need to function properly, and for constraining harmful bacteria and other molecules so they can't get access to (and harm) the rest of the body.

To do these important jobs, your gut relies on healthy intestinal cells and beneficial bacteria, which help manufacture vitamins, absorb minerals, and digest food.

If your gut microbiome is out of whack, or if the problem develops, via irritation or inflammation, into full-blown gut permeability (a.k.a. "leaky gut"), your brain could be in trouble.

Consider this: 60 liters of blood are pumped into your brain every hour, providing oxygen, removing waste products, and delivering nutrients. If that blood is nutrient-deficient, or carrying junk that doesn't belong, it's going to interfere with your brain's function specifically its ability to create necessary neurotransmitters (more about that in a moment.)

As if that weren't enough, a permeable gut can encourage more inflammation in the body, turning all of this into an ongoing cycle.

**Nutrition feeds your mitochondria**

You may remember from high-school biology that mitochondria are the "energy factories" of our cells.

Recent studies suggest that mitochondria play an important role in brain function and cognition and that sub-optimal mitochondria, and mitochondrial diseases, may contribute to mental disorders, including depression.

We don't have a complete picture of what mitochondria need to stay healthy. But we know they need lots of nutrients.

**Nutrition may promote neuroplasticity**

The brain uses nutrients to produce brain-derived neurotrophic factor, or BDNF, a protein that's essential to the central nervous system.

Some research suggests that BDNF could support neuroplasticity the brain's ability to adapt, rewire itself and grow. This would be especially beneficial in recovery from trauma and mental illness.

**What To Do Next**

Depression is overwhelming. Don't try to fix everything at once.

But if you're ready, consider a small, manageable lifestyle-oriented step or two.

First, make sure you're eating, at least a little bit. Depression can do a number on your appetite. But no food means no nutrients. No nutrients means sad brain.

Next, consider one of the following basic steps.

**1. Notice and name:** Before you even start making any changes, get more aware of what you're already doing and feeling.

Try keeping a simple journal for instance, how you're feeling today on a 1-10 scale, what you ate, and any symptoms that you notice.

This will provide a starting point for observing what foods (and other lifestyle factors) might ease or exacerbate your depression (bonus: writing, in general, has been shown to help).

**2. Eat whole foods: Make this as easy as possible:** Find fresh foods that don't take much prep (such as fresh fruits, pre-cut vegetables, or pre-bagged salads).

Get them delivered, either as a grocery delivery or a healthy meal delivery service.

If you have a friend-and-family support network, see if someone is willing to help you with the shopping and cooking.

**3. Avoid or limit the depression-promoting stuff:** What does your food and feelings journal tell you? Do you notice any connections?

*Here are some common ones:*

Alcohol is a nervous system depressant. So, not helpful.

- *Caffeine:* It brings you up then knocks you down. It may also worsen anxiety and insomnia.
- *Sugar:* It may numb the pain or distract you from it for a while, but then it makes you feel worse emotionally and physically especially since it can worsen inflammation.
- *Processed foods:* Some folks notice that they're sensitive to things like preservatives in processed foods.

Some people report that gluten worsens symptoms. Use your journal and see what you notice. Try avoiding gluten-containing foods for a week or so, and observe.

**4. Nurture your gut health:** Keep your gut bacteria and intestinal cells happy. For example:

Eat yogurt and fermented foods such as sauerkraut, kimchi, and pickles, or drink kombucha. These must be in their raw, unpasteurized form to offer live bacteria. You'll find them in the refrigerator section of a well-stocked grocery or health food store.

**Take a probiotic supplement.**

Sip bone broth, a long-simmering stock made with chicken or beef bones. Simply put the bones in a pot, cover with water, and simmer for a loooong time (24 hours is good). The resulting stock contains glycine, which is thought to help with internal wound healing, including in your gut.

Choose meat and dairy that's antibiotic and hormone free (if possible), and comes from a trusted butcher or farm. Buy organic if you can.

Be selective when taking antibiotics, which can kill gut bacteria. If you have to take them, build your belly bacteria back up through fermented foods and probiotics.

Limit refined sugars and grains, which can make gut problems worse.

**5. Supplement with caution:** If there's one thing experts tend to agree on, it's "real food first."

We don't know exactly how specific nutrients work in the context of individual foods, or how they work within the body let alone how they work in pill form.

If you're trying to use supplements to address depression, it's best to work with a doctor and nutrition coach, who can help determine which ones might be right for you.

Supplements such as fish oil, probiotics, B-complex, and/or a good multivitamin could be helpful for depression, but do your homework: Choose a brand with studies supporting its effectiveness for mental health.

Not all supplements are created equal. A low-quality vitamin might contain too low a dose or be hard to absorb.

**Remember The BIG PICTURE**

That's hard when you're depressed. Because your world shrinks to a tiny little black hole.

As much as possible, though, try to focus on the big picture.

***Get outside and get sunlight.*** There's a reason depression is associated with darkness.

***Ask for help.*** Start to find your tribe of helpers. That may include a doctor, a therapist, close supportive friends and family members, a fitness trainer, even a pet.

***Move.*** Depression is immobilizing. Do your best to act against that force by moving whatever you can move, however you can move it.

***Express yourself.*** Draw, write, talk about what you're feeling, howl at the moon. Or, like me, smash a punching bag. Whatever gets the bad stuff out. Don't keep it all in there.

***Depression is difficult.*** But building your personal toolbox of helpful actions can be incredibly empowering. There's no rush. Just start adding in good things to help your body and mind.

# CHAPTER 5

**CONCLUSION**

**Best Depression Treatments**

The best Depression treatments are those that work. There is a wide variety of treatments for Depression and each has its own benefits and draw backs. Treatment of Depression is necessary because it is a serious illness. Without treatment it can only get worse not better.

**Psychotherapy:** This is also called counseling or talk therapy. Some approaches to it are Cognitive/Behavioral, Cognitive, Family Therapy, and psychodynamics. It can help take care of issues relating to sleep, eating, and wrong thinking. There are no known negative effects.

**Holistic Therapy:** The Holistic approach encompasses a variety of treatments. The goal of Holistic medicine is treat the whole person; mind, body, and spirit. Acupuncture, Aroma Therapy, and Chiropractic medicine are just a few of the treatments considered as Holistic. Spirituality or religious experiences can also benefit Depression. There are also no known negative issues with Holistic Therapy.

**Dietary Treatments:** This requires changing the diet to try to improve Depression and other mental health issues. The thinking is that there may be some foods that contain something that might negatively affect your mood. By slowly eliminating then replacing items you might be aware of any food that may be a trigger of your symptoms. The only negative side effect is that your diet could be very restricted.

**Pharmaceutical Treatments:** Anti-depressant medications are beneficial to Depression. They work on the chemicals in the brain either by changing levels of Serotonin and Norepinephrine or making them more bio-available. Anti-depressants come with some very serious side effects not the least of which is suicidal thinking and/or attempts. Suicidal thought seem to be more present in children 21 and under.

**Self-help Treatments:** These treatments are managed by the patient. Meditation and Yoga can be done in a group or alone and benefits Depression. Food can affect mood so it may be the patient only eats certain foods because of the effects some may have on them. Some might plan a special outing or a bubble bath and curling up with a good book. For some chocolate might be used.

Herbal Treatments: A blend of herbs, vitamins and other nutritive substances known to affect mood make up herbal supplements that are usually in capsule form. High quality herbal supplements should be made according to pharmaceutical standards. The metabolic pathways of the ingredients at the molecular level should be studied.

The interaction of the ingredients should be evaluated as well. This guarantees their potency, efficacy, safety, and purity.

Depression is one of the most common conditions in primary care, but is often unrecognized, undiagnosed, and untreated. Depression has a high rate of morbidity and mortality when left untreated. Most patients suffering from depression do not complain of feeling depressed, but rather anhedonia or vague unexplained symptoms. All physicians should remain alert to effectively screen for depression in their patients. There are several screening tools for depression that are effective and feasible in primary care settings. An appropriate history, physical, initial basic lab evaluation, and mental status examination can assist the physician in diagnosing the patient with the correct depressive spectrum disorder (including bipolar disorder). Primary care physicians should carefully assess depressed patients for suicide. Depression in the elderly is not part of the normal aging process. Patients who are elderly when they have their first episode of depression have a relatively higher likelihood of developing chronic and recurring depression. The prognosis for recovery is equal in young and old patients, although remission may take longer to achieve in older patients. Elderly patients usually start antidepressants at lower doses than their younger counterparts.

A surprising number of people will not seek professional help even when it is the right thing to do because they do not like the idea that they require help to manage their issues. If you think seeking help is a weakness, and that only 'weaklings' ever consult professionals, you'll need to decide whether your macho attitude (for that is what that attitude is, regardless of whether you are a man or a woman) is helping or hindering your progress in solving your problems and issues. If your attitude is getting in the way of your growth and health, then you have to decide whether or not it is time to change your attitude. If in your careful estimation self-help will work for you then pursue self-help with determination. First, however, take the necessary time to understand your issues, and explore all of your alternatives for self-help. Avoid risky, extreme, or un-proven methods and 'solutions' that might endanger you or others (if in doubt, consult with a professional). If, however, you've thought it through and have decided that self-help isn't likely to work for you at this time, then seek out professional assistance now. Don't stand in your own way by avoiding professional assistance.

# DISCLAIMER

All the material contained in this book is provided for educational and informational purposes only. No responsibility can be taken for any results or outcomes resulting from the use of this material. While every attempt has been made to provide information that is both accurate and effective, the author does not assume any responsibility for the accuracy or use/misuse of this information.